YOUR KNOWLEDGE HAS VALUE

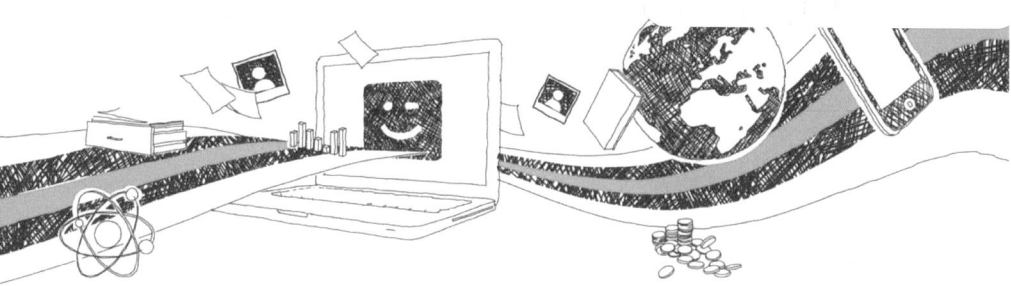

- We will publish your bachelor's and master's thesis, essays and papers

- Your own eBook and book - sold worldwide in all relevant shops

- Earn money with each sale

Upload your text at www.GRIN.com and publish for free

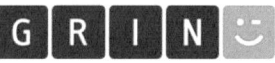

Bibliographic information published by the German National Library:

The German National Library lists this publication in the National Bibliography; detailed bibliographic data are available on the Internet at http://dnb.dnb.de .

This book is copyright material and must not be copied, reproduced, transferred, distributed, leased, licensed or publicly performed or used in any way except as specifically permitted in writing by the publishers, as allowed under the terms and conditions under which it was purchased or as strictly permitted by applicable copyright law. Any unauthorized distribution or use of this text may be a direct infringement of the author s and publisher s rights and those responsible may be liable in law accordingly.

Imprint:

Copyright © 2018 GRIN Verlag
Print and binding: Books on Demand GmbH, Norderstedt Germany
ISBN: 9783668690844

This book at GRIN:

https://www.grin.com/document/419461

Patrick Kimuyu

Theory of Mind Testing in Autistic and Typically Developing Children

GRIN Verlag

GRIN - Your knowledge has value

Since its foundation in 1998, GRIN has specialized in publishing academic texts by students, college teachers and other academics as e-book and printed book. The website www.grin.com is an ideal platform for presenting term papers, final papers, scientific essays, dissertations and specialist books.

Visit us on the internet:

http://www.grin.com/

http://www.facebook.com/grincom

http://www.twitter.com/grin_com

Theory of Mind Testing in Autistic and Typically Developing Children

Name: Patrick Kimuyu

Table of Contents

Introduction 1

Overview of Neural Basis of Theory of Mind in both Autistic and Typically Developing Children 2

Research Methods Used To Examine Theory of Mind in Autistic and Typically Developing Children ... 4

    Shared World Knowledge 4

    Perceiving Social Cues 5

    Interpreting Actions 6

Conclusion 7

References 8

Introduction

Theory of mind has emerged as a philosophical approach with an exceptional social importance. It explains social interactions amongst humans in daily engagements including maintaining emotional intimacy, influencing peers, and acquiring information (Dore, Smith & Lillard, 2015).That level of significance explains why the theory has attracted extensive research attention over the past few decades. Ultimately, traditional research on the theory of mind has revealed the key underpinnings related to the paradigm. It has provided plausible reasons why the theory is essential in constructing mentalistic explanations for human behavior in typically developing individuals. From another perspective, the principle of theory of mind appears to be of paramount significance for social functioning among clinical populations who experience challenges in social interaction. It is useful in explaining complex behaviors that are expressed by individuals with traumatic brain injury (Muller *et al.*, 2010), autism spectrum disorders (Losh, Martin, Klusek, Hogan-Brown & Sideris, 2012), and schizophrenia (Hooker, Bruce, Lincoln, Fisher & Vinogradov, 2011). To examine the theory of mind, researchers have developed several methods, which are based on single task measurements using comprehensive instruments (Blijd-Hoogewys, van Geert, Serra & Minderaa, 2008). However, theorists continue to give conflicting perspectives towards the aspects linked to the theory of mind such as evidence for earlier abilities, task manipulation of the onset of theory of mind, and integrity of false-belief tasks. Therefore, this discussion seeks to provide a focused critical analysis of the research methods used to examine theory of mind, as well as the findings of research in relation to the theory of mind in both typically developing children and those with autism.

Overview of Neural Basis of Theory of Mind in both Autistic and Typically Developing Children

From a critical point of view, the ability to attribute mental states to other people has been found to be age and gender dependent (Calero, Salles, Semelman & Sigman, 2013). However, the development of theory of mind in children is relatively controversial owing to the conflict in different findings. Earlier studies reported that the theory of mind is entirely absent in toddlers (Luo, 2011). Most of these studies were performed in children between 3 and 5 years of age, primarily preschool children. Findings from these studies exhibit lack of consensus on the existence of theory of mind among this age group. However, the same studies reveal that the integral aspects of the theory of mind emerge within this developmental stage (Flavell, 1999; Bartsch & Wellman, 1995). On the other hand, Frith and Frith (2003) posit that children attain theory of mind at the ages of three or four years, a process that has its onset during infancy as early as 18 months. Other studies suggest that children at the age of 5 years still experience instability in theory of mind, especially in developing comprehension in false beliefs (Rai & Mitchell, 2004). This argument is somehow supported by Dumontheil et al. (2010) in a study that found out that children can pass theory of mind tasks at the age of 4 years, but the authors note that significant theory of mind improvements occur in late adolescence. Despite the disagreements on the age at which theory of mind develops, current studies show that theory of mind develops continuously throughout an individual's life, and this comes with remarkable changes (Moran, 2013; Devine & Hughes, 2012; Apperly, 2012).

On an advanced perspective, the development of theory of mind is underpinned by several precursors. It is reported that social environment influences its development in children, gnostic functions, as well as nonverbal communication as expressed through physical and emotional contact between a child and her/his mother. Toddlers show some level of engagement, imitation and empathy; aspects that reflect understanding of another person's mental state (Blair, 2008).

Overall, recent studies have explained how theory of mind develops during childhood. In the initial stages, particularly during infancy and early childhood, children are reported to acquire the essential skills needed for the development of theory of mind in later stages of development. Some of these basic skills include paying attention to other people, as well as imitating or copying them. They also develop a sense of recognizing other people's emotions. Additionally, children begin to recognize their differences from other people, and show some understanding on the causes and consequences of emotions. Finally, it is reported that children start engaging in pretend play whereby they assume to be like other people such as doctor or a teacher (Westby & Robinson, 2014; de Villiers & de Villiers, 2014). In the next stage of development, between 4 and 5 years, typically developing children have been found to develop theory of mind skills in a stepwise manner. First, they understand other people's thoughts and feelings, something that enables them to know that different people act differently to get what they want. Second, they begin to understand 'thinking' of other people. They realize that different people hold different beliefs about a particular subject based on their expectations. Finally, they begin to understand 'false beliefs,' as well as 'hidden feelings' (Wellman & Liu, 2004; Peterson, Wellman & Slaughter, 2012).

However, children with autism exhibit difficulties in developing theory of mind. They have trouble in understanding why others act the way they do. They also have challenges in engaging in conversations, telling a story or socializing with their friends (Kimbi, 2014). One of the unique features that show the difference in theory of mind development between autistic children and typically developing children is the order of understanding 'false beliefs' and 'hidden feelings.' A recent study by Kimbi (2014) showed that children with autism develop understanding of 'hidden feelings' before 'false beliefs' unlike in typically developing children where understanding of 'false belief' emerges first.

Research Methods Used To Examine Theory of Mind in Autistic and Typically Developing Children

With the understanding of how theory of mind develops in both typically developing children and those with autism, it is logical to discuss critically research methods used to examine theory of mind in these populations. In practice, there are three main methods that are used to examine theory of mind; shared world knowledge, interpretation of actions and perceived social cues (Byom & Mutlu, 2013). There are also other emerging methods such as simulated social interaction, which are designed to advance the testing of theory of mind in both physically developing individuals and the clinical populations.

Shared World Knowledge

Shared world knowledge is one of the common methods used to examine theory of mind. It is implicit that an individual's cognition manifests the surrounding world's context (Korkmaz, 2011). For instance, conversation among individuals is based on inferences about thoughts, goals, emotions, and beliefs of those who are involved in any conversation. It is also worth noting that individuals make appropriate responses to their conversational partners through the integration of cues from the context. From this context, any meaningful conversation requires the appropriate use of several aspects. For starters, one requires an appropriate use of prior world knowledge, which may imply the level of comfort of a conversational partner. Second, a conversation requires the existence of the particular goal of interaction. For instance, the completion of a joint task is depended on the availability of the relevant information. Third, a conversation occurs under certain conditions in order to generate useful guesses about the mental state of a conversational partner. Finally, there is need for a clear understanding about the relationship between the conversing parties (Knoblich, Butterfill & Sebanz, 2011).

In the past, several studies have used shared world knowledge to examine theory of mind in both clinical populations and typically developing individuals. For instance, Happé (1994) used text-based tasks, particularly strange stories, to examine theory of mind in autistic and typically developing individuals, and reported that individuals with autism had trouble in using mentalistic explanations to explain strange stories. On the one hand, shared world knowledge is considered as a valuable method for testing theory of mind deficits in clinical populations such as those with autism and traumatic brain injury. However, they impose demands on working memory or linguistic processing, especially verbal and text based tasks (Byom & Mutlu, 2013). An example is the use of stories that require an individual to process the language used in the story, as well as storing information in the working memory. As such, these tasks make this method inappropriate for testing theory of mind in children with autism because they have working memory deficits. Moreover, it is argued that the tasks involved in shared world knowledge method are usually reflective and passive in nature; thus, they can lead to overestimation of theory of mind (Brüne, Abdel-Hamid, Lehmkämper & Sonntag, 2007).

Perceiving Social Cues

Perception of social cues is another method that has been used extensively to examine theory of mind. It is possible to infer the mental state of another individual through perception of social cues. In this context, children's use of facial expressions, vocal cues and gaze cues, are useful parameters that can be used to examine their mental states. This method relies on two main approaches; facial emotion recognition and vocal emotion recognition. It is reported that children with autism have difficulties in identifying mental states using facial affect displays (Peterson, Wellman & Slaughter, 2012). One of the key benefits of this method is that children, as well as adults, have innate abilities to identify emotions with a high degree of accuracy. As such, it is easy to identify theory of mind deficits in both typically developing children and clinical populations, especially those with autism (De Sonneville et al., 2002). Byom and Mutlu (2013) observe that social cues perception tasks have led to advanced understanding of mental state reasoning. However, this method has its limitations. Social cues are considered to have significant limitations in their offline design and they are reflective in nature, aspects that can lead to overestimation of theory of mind in individuals. It is relatively difficult to establish the perception of social cues in daily life interactions due to prolonged thinking time, observation, and combination of isolated social cues (Byom & Mutlu, 2013).

Interpreting Actions

Interpretation of actions is the third method that is used to examine theory of mind. According to Wimmer and Perner (1983), humans as young as 2 years can form expectations about others implies that this ability is useful in testing theory of mind deficits. In this context, several tasks can be used to evaluate the ability of typically developing children and adults to infer mental states from actions or behavior. Based on false belief tasks, researchers have been able to examine theory of mind in both typically developing children and those with autism. For instance, Wimmer and Perner (1983) used reality unknown false belief to evaluate theory of mind in children. The findings of this study showed that typically developing children are able to pass these tasks at 4 years of age. On the other hand, Baron-Cohen et al. (1985) found out that children with autism were not able to pass this task. This method has its potential in testing theory of mind in that; joint action tasks can be used to investigate theory of mind skills in simulated interactions.

Conclusion

Conclusively, it is apparent that theory of mind has attracted immense scientific inquiry. This is attributable to its relevance in treating anxiety disorders and other conditions that affect an individual's cognition such as traumatic brain injury. From a critical review of literature, three main methods: interpretation of actions, perception of social cues, and shared world knowledge have been adopted in evaluating theory of mind in both typically developing individuals and clinical populations, especially those with autism and traumatic brain injury. Each of these methods has its strengths and limitations when applied to test theory of mind in children. However, the emerging simulation-based computational methods seem to provide solutions to some of the drawbacks associated with traditional methods.

References

Apperly I. A. (2012). What is "theory of mind"? Concepts, cognitive processes and individual differences. *Q. J. Exp. Psychol., 65*, 825–839. Doi: 10.1080/17470218.2012.676055

Baron-Cohen, S., Leslie, A. M., & Frith, U. (1985). Does the autistic child have a 'theory of mind'? *Cognition, 21*, 37–46.

Bartsch, K., & Wellman, H. M. (1995). *Children Talk about the Mind.* New York, NY: Oxford University Press.

Blair, R. (2008). Fine cuts of empathy and the amygdala: dissociable deficits in psychopathy and autism. *Q J Exp Psychol., 61*, 157–170.

Brüne, M., Abdel-Hamid, M., Lehmkämper, C., & Sonntag, C. (2007). Mental state attribution, neurocognitive functioning, and psychopathology: what predicts poor social competence in schizophrenia best? *Schizophr. Res., 92*, 151–159.

Byom, L., & Mutlu, B. (2013).Theory of mind: mechanisms, methods, and new directions. *Front Hum Neurosci., 7*, 413.

Calero, C., Salles, A., Semelman, M., & Sigman, M. (2013). Age and gender dependent development of Theory of Mind in 6- to 8-years old children. *Front Hum Neurosci., 7*, 281. doi: 10.3389/fnhum.2013.00281

De Sonneville, L. M. J., Vershoor, C. A., Njiokiktjien, C., Veld, V. H. H., Toorenaar, N., & Vranken, M. (2002). Facial identity and facial emotions: speed, accuracy and processing strategies in children and adults. *J. Clin. Exp. Neuropsychol., 24*, 200–213. Doi: 10.1076/jcen.24.2.200.989

de Villiers, J. G., & de Villiers, P. A. (2014). The role of language in theory of mind development. *Topics in Language Disorders, 34*(4), 313-328.

Devine, R. T., & Hughes, C. (2012). Silent films and strange stories: theory of mind, gender, and social experiences in middle childhood. *Child Dev., 84*, 989–1003. Doi: 10.1111/cdev.12017

Dumontheil, I., Apperly, I. A., & Blakemore, S. (2010). Online usage of theory of mind continues to develop in late adolescence. *Dev. Sci., 13*, 331–338. Doi: 10.1111/j.1467-7687.2009.00888.x

Flavell, J. H. (1999). Cognitive development: children's knowledge about the mind. *Annu Rev Psychol., 50*, 21-45.

Kimbi, Y. (2014). Theory of mind abilities and deficits in autism spectrum disorders. *Topics in Language Disorders, 34*(4), 329-343.

Knoblich, G., Butterfill, S., Sebanz, N. (2011). Psychological research on joint action: theory and data: In B. Ross (Eds), *The Psychology of Learning and Motivation* (pp. 59–101). Burlington, VT: Academic Press.

Korkmaz, B. (2011). Theory of mind and neurodevelopmental disorders of childhood. *Pediatr. Res. 69*(5), 101R–8R.

Luo, Y. (2011). Do 10-month-old infants understand others' false beliefs? *Cognition 121*, 289–298.

Moran, J. M. (2013). Lifespan development: the effects of typical aging on theory of mind. *Behav. Brain Res., 237*, 32–40. Doi: 10.1016/j.bbr.2012.09.020

Peterson, C. C., Wellman, H. M. & Slaughter, V. (2012). The mind behind the message: Advancing theory-of-mind scales for typically developing children, and those with deafness, autism, or asperger syndrome. *Child Development, 83*(2), 469-485.

Rai, R., & Mitchell, P. (2004). Five-year-old children's difficulty with false belief when the sought entity is a person. *J. Exp. Child Psychol., 89*, 112–126. Doi: 10.1016/j.jecp.2004.05.003

Wellman, H. M., & Liu, D. (2004). Scaling theory of mind tasks. *Child Development, 75*, 759-763.

Westby, C. & Robinson, L. (2014). A developmental perspective for promoting theory of mind. *Topics in Language Disorders, 34*(4), 362-383.

Wimmer, H., & Perner, J. (1983). Beliefs about beliefs: representation and constraining function of wrong beliefs in young children's understanding of deception. *Cognition, 13*, 103–128. Doi: 10.1016/0010-0277(83)90004-5

YOUR KNOWLEDGE HAS VALUE

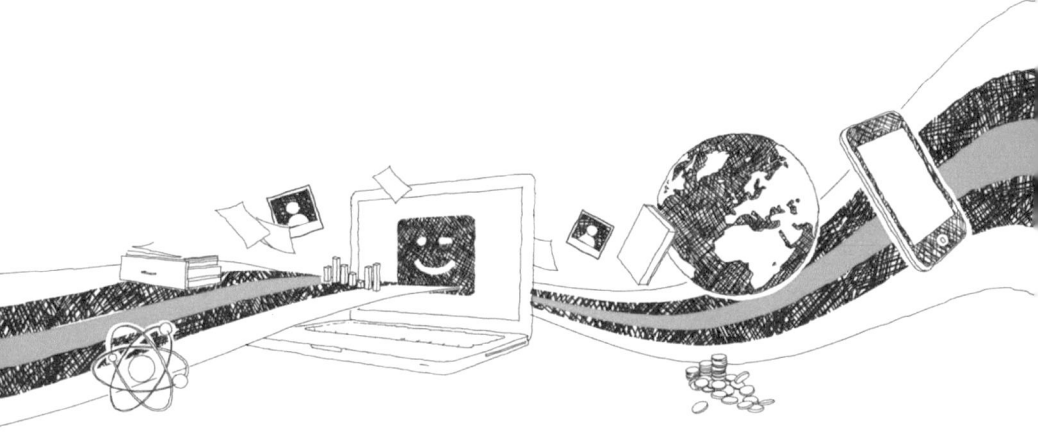

- We will publish your bachelor's and master's thesis, essays and papers

- Your own eBook and book - sold worldwide in all relevant shops

- Earn money with each sale

Upload your text at www.GRIN.com
and publish for free

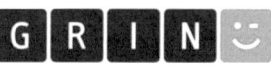